The Effective Nurse Preceptor Handbook

Your Guide to Success

SECOND EDITION

Diana Swihart, PhD, DMin, MSN, CS, RN-BC

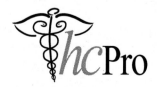

The Effective Nurse Preceptor Handbook: Your Guide to Success, Second Edition
is published by HCPro, Inc.

Copyright ©2007, 2003 HCPro, Inc.

First edition published 2003. Second edition 2007.

ISBN: 978-1-57839-987-1

HCPro, Inc., provides information resources for the healthcare industry.

HCPro, Inc., is not affiliated in any way with The Joint Commission, which owns the
JCAHO and Joint Commission trademarks.

Diana Swihart, PhD, DMin, MSN, CS, RN-BC, Author
Rebecca Hendren, Managing Editor
Lindsey Cardarelli, Associate Editor
Emily Sheahan, Group Publisher
Patrick Campagnone, Cover Designer
Mike Mirabello, Senior Graphic Artist
Jean St. Pierre, Director of Operations
Susan Darbyshire, Art Director
Darren Kelly, Books Production Supervisor
Audrey Doyle, Copyeditor
Sada Preisch, Proofreader

Advice given is general. Readers should consult professional counsel for specific legal,
ethical, or clinical questions.

Arrangements can be made for quantity discounts. For more information, contact

HCPro, Inc.
P.O. Box 1168
Marblehead, MA 01945
Telephone: 800/650-6787 or 781/639-1872
Fax: 781/639-2982
E-mail: *customerservice@hcpro.com*

Visit HCPro at its World Wide Web sites:
www.hcpro.com and *www.hcmarketplace.com*

Contents

About the author

Diana Swihart, PhD, DMin, MSN, CS, RN-BC

Dr. Diana Swihart, a clinical nurse specialist in nursing education at the Bay Pines VA Healthcare System in Bay Pines, FL, has a widely diverse background in many professional nursing arenas, theology, ministry, ancient Near Eastern studies, and archaeology. She is a member of the editorial advisory board for *Advance for Nurses,* Florida edition, and the advisory boards for **The Staff Educator** and **Magnet Status Advisor,** published by HCPro, and the Shared Governance Forum online. She is the author of *Shared Governance: A Practical Approach to Reshaping Professional Nursing Practice,* published by HCPro.

She has published and spoken on a number of topics related to nursing, shared governance, evidence-based practice, competency assessment, education, preceptorships, new employee orientation, servant leadership, work-force grants, and nursing professional development, both locally and nationally.

Dr. Swihart has served as an ANCC Magnet Recognition Program® appraiser and is currently an ANCC accreditation appraiser, the treasurer for the National Nursing Staff Development Organization, and adjunct faculty at South University and Trinity Theological Seminary and College of the Bible distance learning program.

The Effective Nurse Preceptor Handbook

Second Edition

Wearing the preceptor hat

An effective preceptor is a major factor affecting the retention of new nurses. Preceptors are nurses who can talk about difficulties they have met, share insights they have gained, and pass on lessons they have learned by caring for patients in the many arenas of need they encounter each day. The right preceptor can help the new nurse or graduate to overcome the hurdles of new technology, inadequate staffing, complicated medical interventions, and complex diagnoses.

Preceptors facilitate the orientation, growth, and development of nurses who will one day work side by side with them, and who will eventually become their peers, colleagues, and leaders. Staff nurses who precept can connect with new hires, students, and new graduate nurses (preceptees) in ways that no one else can, building trust and responsibility as they gently draw their preceptees into the "real world" of healthcare.

Who really benefits from all of this effort? Patients—and us! Effective nurse preceptorships provide the flexibility for the close, trusting relationships needed to develop preceptees to their fullest potential. The next step in building formal and informal professional nurse preceptorships in your organization is to understand the essential roles, responsibilities, and accountabilities of the preceptor and preceptee within the context of those relationships.

This handbook will provide you with the background necessary to help the new hire, student, new graduate nurse, or novice examine and apply nursing theory and evidence-based practice (EBP) in clinical settings, increasing personal and professional growth, while easing the transition into professional practice.

What is a preceptor?

Preceptors are experienced and competent staff nurses who have received formal training to function in this capacity and who serve as role models and resource people to preceptees. They merge the knowledge, skills, abilities, and roles of both coaches and mentors to help preceptees develop and mature into strong practicing professionals within new or different professional practice environments.

A preceptor is a

- servant leader
- educator/teacher
- coach
- encourager
- socializer

- recordkeeper
- evaluator
- advocate
- role model
- mentor

Preceptors are staff nurses who generally have more work experience and knowledge of the organization and unit, are dedicated to helping other nurses advance in their careers, provide feedback on preceptees' strengths and weaknesses, and offer suggestions for improvement in tasks and behaviors. Preceptors help preceptees balance tasks with work issues (e.g., time management, accepting new responsibilities, adjusting to a new work environment and team, stress management, and how to give and receive constructive criticism).

Other preceptor roles include the following:

- Providing leadership, guidance, and support
- Modeling desired skills and behaviors
- Listening and communicating with empathy and patience
- Providing organization and unit information
- Managing the preceptee's orientation and initial competencies

Essential expectations and responsibilities

If you are to be all of these things, you must be willing to take on the following 12 essential responsibilities:

1. Orient your preceptee to the nursing unit. Begin by introducing yourself to your preceptees and reviewing the orientation, competency assessment, and competency verification processes with them. Talk about yourselves and get to know each other. If you have attended a preceptor workshop that used the *Effective Nurse Preceptor Workbook*, complete the preceptor and preceptee interview together to help you get to know one another. This will help you be more sensitive to the unique concerns and needs of your preceptees and be more successful in meeting the goals of the preceptorships.

- Introduce the preceptee to unit staff members.

- Show the preceptee around, where to put his or her things, and so on.
- Describe the chain of command.
- Talk about what's happening in the unit.
- Be positive—stay with the preceptee.
- Put yourself in his or her position; remember what it was like to be "new."
- Practice whatever you preach.
- Initiate the orientation and competency assessment processes.

2. Facilitate the learning experience. Begin by reflecting on your own behaviors, skills, abilities, and attitudes. Consider what you want to accomplish through the preceptorship, and if you attended a preceptor workshop that used the *Effective Nurse Preceptor Workbook,* complete the preceptor development plan.

Facilitating learning is not the same as learning to give an injection. Facilitating learning in preceptorships is about providing support that will help your preceptee come to work with a positive attitude, practice skills until they are mastered, and develop and model professional behaviors. Your preceptees need your support and encouragement to apply the things you are teaching them during orientation and when verifying initial competencies. They draw on many academic and life experiences to form their beliefs and expectations about what constitutes excellence in nursing. You provide the support, advocacy, parameters, and setting for them to achieve what they have learned.

3. Establish the schedule for your preceptee. Prepare your schedule for the anticipated length of the preceptorship with your preceptee and any input from the unit nurse manager. Discuss any potential scheduling conflicts and ensure that you will spend as much time with the preceptee as possible. Identify a backup preceptor (assistant or substitute, preferably with training/experience as a preceptor) for those shifts or limited times when your schedule conflicts with that of your preceptee. Preceptees should *not* be added to the unit staffing mix until the preceptorship and clinical orientation have been completed. It is the preceptor's role to protect and advocate for the preceptee in such things whenever necessary.

4. Guide your preceptee during clinical practice. You may need to provide direct guidance during the orientation and when verifying initial competencies for the preceptee:

- To demonstrate nursing skills and techniques
- To supervise clinical practice
- To intervene *only* in an emergent situation in which there may be a danger to a patient
- To assess and verify initial competencies

Continuously assess where your preceptees are in the preceptorship. Revise the orientation to reflect their changing needs. Some new nurses are seasoned practitioners and may require only minimal guidance. Student nurses and new nurse graduates often bring life experiences and past professional roles to their clinical positions. Still other preceptees may have difficulty changing methods of practice to reflect their new expectations. Give them respectful guidance.

- Do not assume that preceptees are familiar with the clinical setting or the situation. Discuss what they know before deciding what they need.

- Ask questions to confirm comprehension and perceptions—yours and theirs—and to generate further discussion. Case studies, debriefings, and shared stories are excellent tools for giving directions and encouragement/verifying competency/redirecting behaviors.
- Include explanations as you go. Preceptees respond more positively and effectively when they understand from the onset why they are doing the requested tasks or behaviors.

5. Supervise initial competency assessment and verification during clinical practice. Competency assessment and verification are generally specific to the needs of the preceptee. Make sure you allow your preceptees to assist in deciding what unit-based competencies need to be addressed besides those required for new hires to meet organizational and nursing service goals:

- Select competencies that matter to the new employee or student nurse. Choose assignments that will give the preceptee opportunities to demonstrate those competencies.
- Select the correct verification method (tests/exams, return demonstrations, evidences of daily work, case studies, exemplars, peer reviews, self-assessments, discussion/reflection groups, presentations, mock events/surveys, quality improvement monitors) for each identified competency.
- Clarify the responsibility and accountability of the preceptor, preceptee, and nurse manager in the competency process.
- Implement a preceptee-centered verification process in which the preceptee has choices from among a number of verification methods for the identified competencies.
- Differentiate what is a competency deficit versus what is a compliance issue.

- Promptly and efficiently address any deficits and performance problems with the preceptee as soon as they are identified.

6. Teach new skills and reinforce previous learning. Establish what your preceptees already know or can do; demonstrate the new skills, knowledge, or abilities; have preceptees perform any return demonstrations, if necessary; and evaluate the outcomes when the new knowledge, skill, or ability is applied in practice during the preceptorship.

7. Gradually increase your preceptee's responsibility for patient care. Preceptees often require three to six months, and sometimes as much as a year, to be fully integrated into the culture of the new organization. Orientations usually range from a few days to four to six weeks, depending on the organization and the resources available for new employees. Discuss the amount of time available for the preceptorship with preceptees and nurse managers. Assess preceptees' clinical orientation and competency verification needs and assign increasing responsibilities as they become more proficient and confident in their abilities to practice safely and effectively in their new positions. Help them set priorities, establish daily goals, manage time, delegate appropriately, and communicate professionally with other team members as you gradually introduce new and more challenging patient care assignments.

8. Provide timely feedback to your preceptee regarding all aspects of clinical practice. You must give consistent, fair, honest, and timely verbal and written feedback to your preceptees often. This feedback serves two primary purposes:

- To reinforce positive behavior
- To promptly address inappropriate behaviors

9. Serve as a role model for your preceptee during clinical experiences. This may be your greatest challenge as a preceptor. Subtle techniques that can help you serve as a consistent role model for your preceptees include the following:

- Dress professionally. Maintain clean and appropriate uniforms, if applicable.
- Be prompt and timely, and maintain excellent attendance. Arrive before your preceptee.
- Be prepared for report and participate if applicable.
- Follow nursing service policies and procedures at all times.
- Be courteous and respectful of all team members and leadership at all times, especially when you disagree with their decisions or abilities.
- Stay positive and enthusiastic about professional nursing but realistic in recognizing limitations and areas for improvement.
- Maintain your membership and activities in professional organizations and affiliations.

10. Work closely with nursing faculty/staff development specialists/hospital educators to identify education gaps and learning opportunities. Use your human resources—internal and external stakeholders, clinical educators, advanced practice nurses, pharmacists, biomedical staff, informatics staff, housekeepers, students, college/university partners, community members—to provide more complex and integrated training opportunities. As the preceptor, you will coordinate the preceptees' learning activities with the appropriate resources and verify the preceptees' competencies with patient care outcomes.

11. Plan *specific* learning experiences that correlate with unit competencies and clinical objectives. Ensure that your preceptees have as many opportunities for supervised practice for the wide variety of skills, knowledge, and abilities as they need to be successful in the assigned position and nursing unit. Be particularly careful to verify competencies in any skill with potential patient outcomes that are high-risk (have a high probability of causing potential harm to the patient or preceptee) and time-sensitive (there would be no time to call for help or look up the procedure first). Mock events and return demonstrations are helpful in providing practice and in verifying such competencies.

12. Complete all necessary paperwork related to the preceptorship. Complete preceptor/preceptee interview forms, skills checklists, orientation forms, competency verification forms, feedback, and evaluations in a timely manner. Review all appropriate documents with the preceptee/clinical nurse educator and hospital educator/nurse manager. Maintain careful records in a secure area. Remember, these always have some information that neither you nor your preceptees may want to share with others.

How adults learn

Preceptees come to the preceptoring relationship as adult learners seeking to increase their knowledge, skills, and abilities in new and changing professional practice settings. The preceptee's goal is to successfully complete his or her orientation and competency verification periods. The preceptor is a role model who possesses the knowledge and experience necessary to help the preceptee meet that goal.

Effective facilitation occurs when preceptors understand adult learning principles and encourage preceptees to be creative and independent in meeting their orientation and competency requirements, to think critically, and to formulate their own professional strengths and abilities. Preceptors establish rapport with preceptees by acknowledging their lived experiences, thoughts, and feelings about matters related to patient assignments, activities, policies, and other concerns, and encouraging them to ask questions/express personal viewpoints.

When preceptors are facilitating the learning process with preceptees, there are several major questions to consider:

1. What is to be learned from the preceptee's assignment or experience?
2. What knowledge/skills/abilities are "need to know" versus "nice to know"?
3. How is the information to be used or implemented?
4. How and when is the learning to be accomplished?
5. How is the learning to be communicated/documented?
6. How is the learning to be evaluated?
7. How can the preceptor facilitate the learning?

Accessing information through learning styles

To understand how to teach others, you must have an understanding of the variety of ways that people learn. The "learning style inventory test" that follows will provide some insight into how preceptees prefer to access information. The best learning and application to practice occur when all learning styles are used together. Complete the test and then score the test using the "scoring procedures" guide.

Are you a visual, auditory, or kinesthetic (tactile) learner? Do you see the implications that each learning style may have for how preceptees access information during the orientation and competency verification process?

Learning Style Inventory Test

To gain a better understanding of yourself as a learner, you need to evaluate the way you prefer to learn or process information. By doing so, you will be able to develop strategies that will enhance both your learning and teaching potential.

This 24-item survey is not timed. Answer each question as honestly as you can.

Place a ✓ on the appropriate line after each statement.

	Often	Sometimes	Seldom
1. Can remember more about a subject through the lecture method, with information, explanations, and discussion.			
2. Prefer information to be written on the chalkboard, with the use of visual aids and assigned readings.			
3. Like to write things down or to take notes for visual review.			
4. Prefer to use posters, models, actual practice, and some activities in class.			
5. Require explanations of diagrams, graphs, or visual directions.			
6. Enjoy working with my hands or making things.			
7. Am skillful with, and enjoy developing and making, graphs and charts.			
8. Can tell whether sounds match when presented with pairs of sounds.			
9. Remember best by writing things.			
10. Can understand and follow directions on maps.			
11. Do better at academic subjects by listening to lectures and tapes.			
12. Play with coins or keys in pockets.			

	Often	Sometimes	Seldom
13. Learn to spell better by repeating the words out loud than by writing the word on paper.	_____	_____	_____
14. Can better understand a news article by reading about it in the paper than by listening to the radio.	_____	_____	_____
15. Chew gum, smoke, or snack during studies.	_____	_____	_____
16. Feel the best way to remember is to picture it in my head.	_____	_____	_____
17. Learn spelling by "finger spelling" words.	_____	_____	_____
18. Would rather listen to a good lecture or speech than read about the same material in a textbook.	_____	_____	_____
19. Am good at working and solving jigsaw puzzles and mazes.	_____	_____	_____
20. Grip objects in hands during learning period.	_____	_____	_____
21. Prefer listening to the news on the radio rather than reading about it in the newspaper.	_____	_____	_____
22. Obtain information on an interesting subject by reading relevant materials.	_____	_____	_____
23. Feel very comfortable touching others, hugging, handshaking, and so on.	_____	_____	_____
24. Follow oral directions better than written ones.	_____	_____	_____

Scoring Procedures

Please insert the following point values on the line next to the corresponding item. Add the points in each column to obtain the total preference scores under each heading.

Often = 5 points   Sometimes = 3 points   Seldom = 1 point

Visual		Auditory		Tactile	
No.	Pts.	No.	Pts.	No.	Pts.
2.		1.		4.	
3.		5.		6.	
7.		8.		9.	
10.		11.		12.	
14.		13.		15.	
16.		18.		17.	
19.		21.		20.	
22.		24.		23.	
Total VPS		Total APS		Total TPS	

VPS = Visual Preference Score
APS = Auditory Preference Score
TPS = Tactile Preference Score

If your VSP total was highest, you are a VISUAL learner.
Advice: Be sure that you look at all study materials. Use charts, maps, videos, notes, and flash cards. Practice visualizing or picturing words/concepts in your head. Write out everything for frequent and quick visual review.

If your APS total was highest, you are an AUDITORY learner.
Advice: You may wish to use tape recordings. Tape lectures to help you fill in the gaps in your notes. But do listen and take notes, and review those notes frequently. Sit somewhere in the lecture hall or classroom where you can hear well. After you have read something, summarize it and recite it aloud.

If your TPS total was highest, you are a TACTILE learner.
Advice: Trace words as you are saying them. For facts that must be learned, you should write them out several times. Keep a supply of scratch paper for this purpose. Taking and keeping lecture notes will be very important. Make study sheets.

Precepting/teaching effectiveness

A basic understanding of policies used within the organization is required of nursing students and new employees. A **visual** learner may be able to read the policies and understand them. An **auditory** learner may need to have the policies read out loud and discussed. A **tactile** learner may have to actually implement the policies—in other words, do something—to fully grasp the policies.

Select teaching strategies that engage all the senses to maximize retention of information and learning.

Teaching strategies in the three learning domains

There are three learning domains: the cognitive domain, the psychomotor domain, and the affective domain. Each time you begin a teaching session, you must consider the domain in which you are teaching.

The **cognitive domain** focuses on preceptees' knowledge and intellectual skills. Teaching strategies include lectures, presentations, tests, case studies, and written materials. Test retention with objective and subjective test items (e.g., ask the preceptee to calculate a drug dose [objective] and choose an accurate pain description on a patient pain scale [subjective]). The cognitive domain addresses three instructional levels: fact, understanding, and application.

- **Fact:** Preceptees are asked to recall information; learning objectives use verbs such as *define, match,* and *list.*
- **Understanding:** Preceptees join two or more concepts; learning objectives use verbs such as *describe, explain,* and *contrast.*
- **Application:** Preceptees merge two or more concepts and apply

this knowledge to a new situation; learning objectives use verbs such as *apply, demonstrate,* and *illustrate.*

The **psychomotor domain** focuses on preceptees' skills and physical abilities. Teaching strategies include performance skill-testing, mock events, quality improvement monitors, return demonstrations, and evidence of daily work. The psychomotor domain addresses three instructional levels: imitation, practice, and habit.

- **Imitation:** Preceptees complete a return demonstration of skill, either under direct supervision of the preceptor or with evidence of daily work (e.g., passing a medication and accurately charting it as evidenced by the chart review and patient's report); learning objectives use verbs such as *follow directions, initiate,* and *carry out.*

- **Practice:** Preceptees have the opportunity to repeat the sequence of events in any procedure as often as needed to build proficiency without direct supervision; learning objectives use verbs/phrases such as *repeat, perform,* and *go through the motion.*

- **Habit:** Preceptees perform the identified skill in twice the time it takes the preceptor to perform it; learning objectives use verbs/phrases such as *perform rapidly, fit action to a new situation,* and *complete smoothly and efficiently.*

The **affective domain** focuses on preceptees' emotionally based behaviors. Teaching strategies include reflective exemplars, self-assessments, discussions, storytelling, and peer reviews. Learning objectives use verbs such as *accept, challenge, defend, dispute, judge, praise, question, support,* and *share.* The affective domain addresses three instructional levels: awareness, distinction, and integration.

Creating a climate for learning

Establish a learning climate on the nursing unit that will help you implement the adult learning principles.

Physical challenges

The unit environment has to be consciously shaped to maximize personal interaction and learning. There must be suitable places for quiet reading, one-on-one discussions, small class settings, and practice space for demonstrations using mannequins or models.

Emotional challenges

The creation of a nonthreatening emotional climate is a little more challenging and will take a little more time for you to achieve. The emotional climate will serve as a comfort zone, where everyone understands that every person's views are valued and respected as equal. How each member of the unit staff speaks to others in the group is important, as is full unit participation. One way to test the emotional climate is to encourage your preceptee to bring up subjects or ideas for discussion during staff meetings.

Validating competency

Competency is the goal of the precepting process. Competency-based orientations initiate competency assessment and verification processes for preceptees during the orientation.

Competencies can be measured against well-developed professional standards published by respected organizations (e.g., state boards of nursing, professional nursing organizations, or The Joint Commission). They can be improved through training and development. Therefore,

Tender Greens
1640 Camino del Rio North
San Diego, CA 92108
Tel.

Server: Benjamin   01/05/2017
Cashier: Kathryn
Ruth/1   5:26 PM
Guests 0

                               #10296

Steak Salad   12.00

Subtotal   12.00
Tax   0.93

Total   12.93

VISA   12.93
  Auth:092635

 + Tip: _____

 = Total: _____

X_____

Balance Due   0.00

"Eat food. Not too much. Mostly plants."
              -Michael Pollan
              tendergreens.com

          --- Check Closed ---

one of the major roles of preceptors is to assess and verify competencies during orientation.

Orientation and verifying competency processes

Competency-based orientations offer numerous advantages for preceptorships. They give clear guidelines regarding competency expectations and can decrease the amount of time spent in orientation for more experienced/skilled preceptees, such as those who have worked in the organization/nursing department but recently transferred from another department or unit. Preceptees who have difficulty completing their initial competencies are quickly identified. Preceptors can review the competency assessment and verification form with preceptees to provide timely feedback on progress and remediate/restructure their clinical experiences to address those deficits or problem areas.

The three important elements of competency-based orientations are as follows:

1. **Technical competence.** This is the most familiar and objective skill domain. Elements are traditionally found on checklists, and competency is measured by direct observation of psychomotor tasks. Efficiency components are often added to assess advanced competency.

   • Start an IV and manage the equipment properly.
   • Draw blood from an arterial line.
   • Verify accuracy of data transfer.
   • Identify problematic lab values and take appropriate actions.
   • Respond to STAT orders within 30 minutes.

2. **Interpersonal competence.** This skill domain refers to the effective use of interpersonal communication when working with others. These competencies, too, are often found on checklists and are measured by direct observation of interactions and behaviors that consistently convey caring and courteous attitudes.

   - Greet staff, patients, and families with warmth and genuineness.
   - Call the patient by his or her preferred name.
   - Display proper phone etiquette.
   - Anticipate patient and family anxiety and offer information, reassurance, and comfort as appropriate.
   - Work cooperatively with team members.

3. **Critical thinking (or decision-making) competence.** This skill domain addresses preceptees' abilities to apply principles of critical thinking, problem solving, and decision-making to EBP. To measure competencies in this skill domain, preceptors must be more creative in their verification methods. Competencies are predicated on preceptees' abilities to recognize problems, identify alternative actions, anticipate outcomes, and make choices based on the most current best practices. Asking questions helps them get beneath the surface of problems, generate more questions, and increase the number of possible solutions.

   - Ask "why" questions.
   - Look for patterns and trends; be open to possibilities.
   - View events as part of a larger whole.
   - Use intuition and "hunches" when problem solving.
   - Seek advice.

QUESTIONS TO PROMOTE CRITICAL THINKING

Preceptorships provide a safe environment during orientation for preceptees to explore the challenging problems found in complex healthcare systems. Guided questions can stimulate critical thinking and enhance preceptees' decision-making skills.

- Given these lab results, how will you change your nursing care plan?
- How will you prioritize your care today?
- What alternative nursing measures would work in this situation?
- What else could be causing your patient's symptoms?
- How will you determine the effectiveness of that intervention?
- How will you document your patient's outcomes related to that treatment?

Do not confuse personality traits or characteristics with competency. They are not performance indicators. The following is a list of some common traits that you should not use to evaluate competency:

• Cooperative	• Conforms to policies	• Codependent
• Assertive	• Is a team player	• Flexible
• Aggressive	• Shows initiative	• Passive
• Committed	• Decisive	• Creative

Preceptors frequently need to check their perceptions with their preceptees before making a final decision regarding competency levels of knowledge, skills, or abilities in any skill domain, to ensure objectivity rather than subjectivity.

Providing feedback

Your preceptee needs daily feedback on the things he or she is doing well, areas in which additional work is needed, and progress toward goals.

Feedback must be specific, factual, descriptive, clearly understood by the preceptor and preceptee, timed to be most useful, sensitive to the preceptor and preceptee, constructive, and directed at behavior rather than personality traits. Whenever possible, provide positive feedback. When necessary, provide constructive feedback. Avoid giving negative feedback if at all possible. Complete the evaluation form you use in your facility at each agreed-upon time interval (e.g., every week during the preceptorship) and at the termination of the preceptoring relationship. When giving feedback, do the following:

- Describe specifically what was observed—who, what, when, where, and how.
- Avoid generalizing or making assumptions.
- Relate how the observed behavior or actions made you feel.
- Suggest an alternative behavior or action.

Continuous feedback allows preceptors to

- motivate and positively reinforce learning
- diagnose the nature and extent of any problem areas
- offer constructive criticism when needed

- identify areas for remediation
- determine the effectiveness of the learning activities

Guidelines for providing effective feedback

Positive feedback affirms or reinforces the preceptee's clinical performance. For example, the preceptor observes the preceptee admit a new patient and document his or her assessment in accordance with established policies and procedures. The preceptor then tells the preceptee, "Congratulations! Your patient admission was done perfectly." Result for the preceptee:

- Affords feelings of success
- Enhances motivation for learning
- Reinforces desired performance

Negative feedback inhibits or modifies the preceptee's clinical performance. For example, the preceptor sees that the preceptee's admitting documentation is incomplete and states, "You did not document that admission correctly." Result for the preceptee:

- Tends to discourage and demoralize
- Limits or reduces motivation for learning
- Tends to focus on what not to do

It is important for preceptors to practice giving constructive feedback whenever preceptees need to correct or improve their performance.

Constructive feedback, like negative feedback, is intended to modify performance but, like positive feedback, conveys its message with supportive language. For example, the preceptor tells the preceptee,

"I reviewed your admission documentation and found that almost all of the important areas were well documented. Because these areas were covered so well, I was surprised to find that no entries were made for the patient's allergies or medication history. Could you tell me why these were omitted?" Result for the preceptee:

- Enables him or her to experience at least partial success
- Maintains motivation for learning
- Reinforces desired performance and corrects unsatisfactory performance

B.E.E.R. feedback method

One technique for creating effective feedback is to use the following four-step model for criticizing and correcting behavior and performance problems.

This model is based on a process that involves asking yourself questions about your preceptee's behavior. Remember the acronym "B.E.E.R.":

B: Behavior—What is the employee doing or not doing that is unacceptable?

E: Effect—Why is the behavior unacceptable? How does it hurt productivity, bother others, and so on?

E: Expectation—What do you expect the employee to do or not do to change?

R: Result—What will happen if the employee changes (positive tone) or this behavior continues (negative tone)?

Comparison examples of applied feedback

Once you have formulated your feedback, use the following rules as guidance on giving effective feedback to your preceptee.

Use descriptive rather than evaluative terms. Always make a conscious effort to describe both positive and negative behaviors.

For example, the preceptor observes the preceptee greeting the patient correctly, giving her name, and stating that she will be her nurse for the day. However, she was not wearing her name tag. Evaluative feedback: "Your name tag is missing, and the manager won't like it!" Descriptive feedback: "You greeted that patient according to the unit guidelines. Can you think of anything that would help your patient remember you?" Have the preceptee use critical thinking to discover the problem.

Be specific rather than general in comments. For example, the preceptee learned how to successfully initiate IV therapy last week. General anecdotal feedback: "IV initiation skills acceptable." Specific anecdotal feedback: "Preceptee initiated three IV starts with a single attempt each time; aseptic technique used; patient stated that process was comfortable."

Focus on your preceptee's behavior, rather than on his or her personality. For example, the preceptee has been consistently late for the patient report at the beginning of the shift and disrupts the shift report when he does get there. The rest of the staff members have complained to the preceptor about the rude, disruptive behavior, saying the preceptee is inconsiderate. Personality-based feedback: "You have been very inconsiderate of the other staff members. They don't like you interrupting report." Behavior-based feedback: "You have been arriving at report late this week. Is there a problem arriving on time? When a staff member is late, it disrupts the flow of the report, and items may be missed. What can you do to ensure that you are here on time?"

Focus on sharing information, rather than giving advice. For example, a patient's dressing change is due. Giving advice: "I think you (the preceptee) should do Mrs. Jones' dressing now. She is scheduled for therapy at 3 p.m." Sharing information: "I just got a call from therapy; Mrs. Jones is scheduled for 3 p.m. Is there anything she needs to have done before her appointment?"

Feedback should be well timed. For example, the preceptor observes a mistake in the preceptee's transcription of a physician's order. Poorly timed feedback: "You made a mistake and need to correct it," said while at the nurses' station and in front of the unit clerk. Well-timed feedback: Preceptor removes the chart to the break room and tells the preceptee privately, "You made a mistake and need to correct it."

Give your preceptee enough time to accept the feedback prior to making a plan that will involve change in behavior. For example, the preceptor observes that the preceptee consistently fails to listen to all areas of the chest when doing a respiratory assessment. Impatient preceptor feedback: "You consistently fail to listen to all areas of the posterior and anterior chest when doing your respiratory assessment. What are you going to do about it?" Patient preceptor feedback: "You consistently fail to listen to all areas of the posterior and anterior chest when doing your respiratory assessment. Please review the assessment process in your text and get back to me tomorrow about how you can use this information to improve your skills."

Avoid giving the impression that you and other staff members are "ganging up" on your preceptee. An example is when staff members complain that the preceptee is taking too much time to complete his or her charting. "Ganging-up" approach: "The staff and I feel that you are spending too much time with patients and not enough time completing your charting." Alternative approach: "I have observed you spending a lot of time with patients, but your documentation has not been complete. How can you complete your charting and still spend needed time with your patients?"

Performance evaluation process

Performance evaluations facilitate preceptees' learning and successful transition into their new practice settings. They should be affirming and future-oriented. As each required competency is successfully demonstrated, tell your orientee that an objective has been completed. Review the documentation form each day and check off the day's accomplishments. This exercise helps your orientee identify progress and feel successful.

It is also important to communicate to your orientee the areas that need further experience or improvement. Be direct and address negatives first. Do not sandwich negatives between two positives; that approach dilutes the effectiveness of both. Do not be apologetic about constructive criticism. As a preceptor, you have both a right and a responsibility to require good performance.

Collaborate with your orientee to develop a plan to improve these areas. Areas for improvement must be discussed as they are identified.

Also, keep the manager updated on any areas that are failing to progress as expected.

End-of-orientation evaluation

There should be *no* surprises at the end of the orientation or at the close of the formal preceptorship program. Select an appropriate setting to review and discuss the final performance evaluation summary.

- Select a quiet, controlled environment without interruptions.
- Maintain a relaxed but professional atmosphere.
- Put the preceptee at ease.
- Review specific examples of both positive and negative behaviors, activities, and attitudes.
- Discuss future needs and goals.

Express confidence in the preceptee's ability to do the work (unless there is good reason not to, which you should have already addressed in previous feedback sessions). *Do not* be hesitant in your encouragement of the preceptee's abilities as appropriate.

- Be sincere and constructive in both praise and criticism.
- Ask the preceptee how the preceptor (you) and clinical educator/nurse manager can improve the preceptorship.

Initiate the peer relationship for preceptees and communicate this change in status to unit team members. Celebrate their transition into their new roles with a recognition ceremony, certificate of completion, or lunch, for example. Use any strategy to commemorate preceptees' change of status and welcome them to the team.

Confronting reality shock

One of the major problems for healthcare institutions is the loss of new staff during the first six months of their employment. This group is made up of new graduates as well as seasoned professionals who are disillusioned with the modern healthcare environment. This disillusionment is commonly known as "reality shock."

New nurses enter their assigned practice settings eager to begin their new jobs, to meet their new colleagues, and to accept their new challenges. They complete orientation and their initial competency verifications without difficulty. Their preceptors ease the transition into practice and teach them everything they need to be successful. Then, three months to a year later, disillusionment sets in. The preceptee realizes that the new healthcare environment is flawed.

There are four phases to reality shock.

1. **Honeymoon phase.** Preceptees are happy to be in their clinical rotations/finished with school/starting a new job. They perceive the new practice setting and their new coworkers positively, or through "rose-colored glasses." When asked, they may say, "Everything is wonderful!" During this phase, preceptees are actively focused on developing their own skills, mastering work routines, and meeting new people.

2. **Shock phase.** Preceptees begin to encounter weaknesses, discrepancies, and inconsistencies in the work environment and their new colleagues:

- Coworkers with weaknesses—disorganized, tardy, or inattentive to duties
- Lack of supplies, poor equipment maintenance, communication breakdown, or other obstacles to providing excellent, or "textbook," nursing care
- Potential inconsistencies in expected professional nursing behaviors
- Any situation that can cause frustration, anger, embarrassment, or disillusionment, such as being humiliated by another nurse or physician

3. **Recovery phase.** Preceptees begin to perceive the realities of the professional practice environment with a balanced view of both negative and positive aspects. They establish expectations that are consistent for all coworkers. The perspective that not all healthcare providers conform uniformly to the professional or organizational standards for conduct must come from within the work setting. Once they achieve this, preceptees recognize their own fallibility. Their sense of humor may return during this phase.

4. **Resolution phase. Caution!** Preceptees may adopt less-than-ideal values or beliefs to resolve the conflicts of values and find ways to "fit in" with their new coworkers. Preceptors must help them retain the positive aspects of both values and belief systems—those taught at school and those held by practicing nurses.

How do you, as the preceptor, work within each of these phases to ensure that reality shock does not lead to resignation or adoption of poor values?

Ways to assist preceptees through workplace acclimation
Honeymoon
- Develop the initial bonds between preceptors and preceptees, created by a mutual sense of trust, respect, and honor.
- Harness their enthusiasm for learning new skills and routines.
- Be realistic, but do not stifle their enthusiasm.
- Introduce them to new staff and coworkers.

Shock
- Anticipate that preceptees may experience some dissatisfaction with new positions/peers/employers.
- Listen attentively.
- Model the ideals of professional nurses.
- Help preceptees find appropriate supplies and functional equipment when needed.
- Provide opportunities to vent frustrations in a constructive manner.

Recovery
- Always treat preceptees kindly.
- Help them view situations realistically.
- Ask them to keep a journal of improvements they would like to suggest and what outcomes they expect or would like to see.
- Help them recognize positive aspects of their current work settings, as well as areas where improvements might be made.
- Ease them into their roles and responsibilities; do not release preceptees to take full patient assignments until ready.
- Protect them in times of adversity.
- Always speak kindly about nurses and other healthcare providers.
- Help preceptees regain their sense of humor.

Resolution

- Identify and manage any conflicts and confusions that persist.
- Assist them in constructive and creative problem solving.
- Describe mechanisms and processes available to resolve perceived problems or confusion.
- Give simple, easy-to-follow directions for tasks.
- Help them combine the best aspects of their prior school or work expectations with their current work situations.
- Caution: Help preceptees retain the positive aspects of their nursing values/belief systems from school and from the practicing nurses.

It is very important that you recognize when your preceptee is in the shock phase. Continue with the open communication pattern already developed. To help your preceptee move toward the recovery phase, a balanced view of the workplace must be presented. Here again, open, honest communication regarding the nursing unit must be held. The expression of genuine feelings and your own stories and real-life anecdotes about situations you have faced, actions contemplated, and outcomes achieved show your preceptees that they, too, can overcome obstacles to professional practice.

Letting go

"Letting go" begins with the welcome. Part of the planning for every preceptorship is the termination. Most organizations have time-limited orientations and clinical periods for competency assessments and verifications for new hires. New-graduate nurses may require additional time, which is negotiated during the feedback sessions as the orientation unfolds.

There are several things to watch out for that indicate that preceptees are ready for the increased responsibilities of a staff nurse and disengagement (letting go) from the preceptorship:

- Evidence that preceptees will not miss important tasks related to the staff nurse role
- Demonstration that they can use past clinical experiences and apply them to current ones
- Recognition of their own limitations of knowledge or skills
- Evidence of critical thinking skills in the questions they ask
- Actively seeking more challenging experiences and greater autonomy in assignments

Keys for successful disengagement

Disengagement from a preceptorship opens the door for mentoring. Movement toward a peer role and potential mentorship requires three keys to be successful:

- Set expectations for all future performance, outlining the steps needed for all performance activities.
- Motivate preceptees by focusing on strengths, releasing preceptees' potential within the organization.
- Help preceptees find their "best fit" within the unit and organization.

Consider celebrating the transition from preceptor to peer to mentor. Bringing tangible closure to the preceptorship can act as a rite of passage into the new staff nurse role with great expectations and equal measures of humor and resolution. As a preceptor, you did your best. Now let your now former preceptee begin to do his or her best.

31

FINAL EXAM

1. A learning style inventory test reveals that your preceptee is a kinesthetic/tactile learner. Which of the following would likely be the most effective way to teach him or her about the unit's admission database?

   a. Give the preceptee a printout of instructions with which he or she can follow along
   b. Let the preceptee enter sample patient data into the database as you explain it
   c. Use a PowerPoint slide presentation to walk your preceptee through the process
   d. All of the above

2. What are the three skill-based domains of learning?

   a. Psychomotor, cognitive, affective
   b. Visual, auditory, tactile
   c. Imitation, practice, and habit
   d. None of the above

3. The author describes a unit's emotional climate for learning as "a comfort zone, where everyone understands that every person's views are valued and respected equally." What way does the author suggest you test the emotional climate for learning on your unit?

   a. Conduct an anonymous poll of unit staff
   b. Let your preceptee introduce him- or herself to the other unit team members
   c. Ask your manager to conduct a staff evaluation
   d. Encourage your preceptee to bring up a subject or an idea for discussion during a staff meeting

4. Which of the following could you observe to verify, or measure, a preceptee's technical competence?

   a. The way your preceptee draws blood from an arterial line
   b. Your preceptee's greeting technique when taking on a new patient
   c. Your preceptee's ability to be on time for report
   d. The number of times your preceptee uses critical thinking to solve problems

5. Competency consists of what three elements?

   _____
   _____
   _____

6. Giving daily feedback to your preceptee allows you to do which of the following:
   a. Motivate and positively reinforce learning
   b. Diagnose the nature and extent of any problems
   c. Determine the effectiveness of the learning experience
   d. All of the above

7. What is the significance of asking questions?

   _____

   _____

   _____

8. During the end of the orientation evaluation, you mention to your preceptee that since the first day of orientation his or her discharge documentation has been incomplete. What fundamental rule of the final evaluation have you forgotten?

   _____

   _____

   _____

9. Which of the following does the author suggest is an effective way to communicate the preceptee's change of status once the preceptorship is over?
   a. A recognition ceremony
   b. A certificate of completion
   c. A lunch with other staff
   d. All of the above

10. The best way to prevent a new nurse from resigning due to "reality shock" is by establishing clear, open communication with him or her during the first of the four phases of workplace acclimation. The name of that first phase is:
    a. The shock phase
    b. The recovery phase
    c. The honeymoon phase
    d. The resolution phase

ANSWERS TO THE FINAL EXAM

1. B
2. A
3. D
4. A
5. Technical competence, interpersonal competence, and critical thinking/decision-making competence
6. D
7. This helps preceptors and preceptees get beneath the surface of problems, generate more questions, and increase the number of possible solutions.
8. There should be no surprises during the final evaluation. Instead, it should be a summary of the daily feedback you have been giving to your orientee.
9. D
10. C

CERTIFICATE OF COMPLETION

This is to certify that

_____

has read and successfully passed the final exam for

The Effective Nurse Preceptor Handbook: Your Guide to Success, Second Edition

_____

Robert Stuart
Senior Vice President/Chief Operating Officer